I0018194

Introduction to Machine Learning Through Poetry

Analogy: The Fruit Vegetation

The Transdisciplinary and Interdisciplinary School

Climate Change, Yeesho Poetry et Poesie

By Yeeshtdevisingh Hosanee

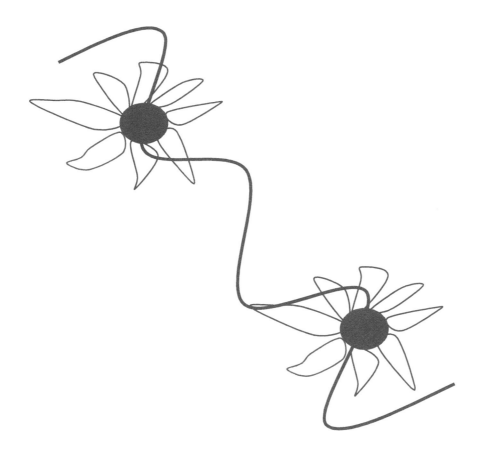

Copyright

© 2025 Hosanee, Yeeshtdevisingh

Title: Introduction to Machine Learning Through Poetry, Analogy: The Fruit Vegetation, The Transdisciplinary and Interdisciplinary School, Climate Change, Yeesho Poetry et Poesie

First Edition: 2025

Publication Date: 01/03/2025

Author, Cover Creator and Illustrator: Yeeshtdevisingh Hosanee

Imprint: Independent Publishing Network, UK

Paperback ISBN: 978-1-83654-735-8

eBook ISBN: 978-1-83654-736-5

Book Series: The Transdisciplinary and Interdisciplinary School

Book Series Number: 1

Book deposited to the UK National Library.

To the Readers

This book, designed in the form of poetry, draws a connection between art and science. Humans possess many tools provided by science. However, with their faculties of calculation, decision-making, creativity, and humor, they still embody the art of nature.

Climate change is becoming an important aspect of our life. Whereas humans' creativity needs to excel through innovation of technologies, machine learning through Artificial Intelligence (AI) concepts requires electrical energy from our world.

Machine Learning (ML) is about learning the environment of the machines. The latter can be computers or smartphones. Humans also learn in a similar way to them. They learn from their environments, finding patterns and construct new things. However, ML happens inside a computer in the digital space, whereas humans learn from a physical environment space.

Humans are the sole species in world to connect dots from physical and digital, vice versa. Understanding how machine learns, can help them to prevent bias and decide when not to use machines to rescue the planet.

As much as innovation is important, climate change, humans and AI need to align. The best way to show their alignment is by using poetry to connect them in an interdisciplinary and transdisciplinary way.

This book reminds us that humans have an identity through all the evolutions of planet Earth, so that Generation Z and Alpha can reclaim these foundations in their leadership.

In this book, the fruit vegetation is used as an analogy to show how cultivation of crops and fruits lead us to the same behaviour as machine learning. The better the cultivation, the better the crops and fruits.

Table of Contents

Poem 1: The Vegetation

Vegetation, a process to cultivate,

Vegetables and fruits interlace,

Assets for the farmer to mitigate,

A sale to a business market as a merchant await,

And merchant's customer awakes.

Vegetation, covered or uncovered,

By greenhouse tent, bewildered,

The farmers' responsibilities unsupervised,

As weather pattern are predicted.

In farmhouse without greenhouse tent covered.

The farmers in a supervised model,

Progressively look at the weather,

And pest challenges unveiled,

Dangers, handled differently echoes,

in uncovered and covered greenhouse scenarios,

By supervised and unsupervised vegetation,

Similar to ML supervised and unsupervised model,

The former, monitors, the latter, less hobble.

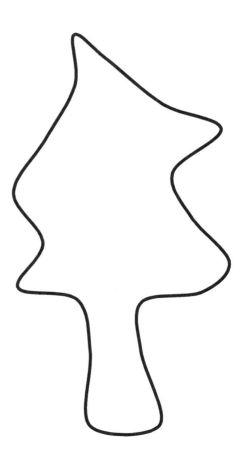

5

Poem 2: The Digital Software

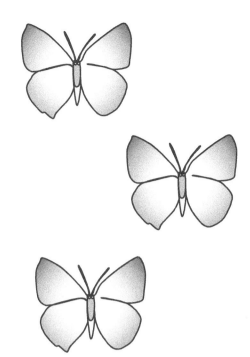

A software, a digital tool

Act like an electric pot suite,

Boiling food noodles curl.

The noodles, are the data,

To the software drama.

Software boils the data,

Present it to computer users' diva,

Akin to food noodles in eaters' plate plea.

A software needs data inputs,

Like the pot's ingredients are inputs,

Vegetables, meat, added to the pot view.

Software's Inputs, encoded and decoded,

Into digital information, ready for moulded,

By a user, who is devoted to a computer software.

Pot's inputs, encoded and decoded,

Into boiled meat noodles, ready for moulded,

By a person, eater, who is devoted to noodle pot.

Software, alike pot, boiled inputs,

By decoding them, like pull ups,

Encoding them in the boiled loops,

Presenting a person, the output.

Their similar behaviours, exemplified,

From inputs, boiled, outputs, mechanised.

Their differences, compartmentalized,

Software, lives in digital designed,

The pot, lives in the physical designed.

The digital designed, moves flows,

Of inputs, boiled, outputs in digital rows.

The physical designed, moves flows,

Of inputs, boiled, outputs in real-life rows.

Poem 3: The Digital Data

Digital data, a meaningless information,

Collected by digital medium transmission,

Collected for physical communication.

A value "1234" is meaningless,

Its interpretation is countless.

Digital medium transmits the value invisibly.

Digital software decodes the value contextually,

From valueless to encode into valuable information quest.

"1234" contextually could be a phone number desk.

"1234" could also become a student ID vest.

Explicit and implicit index, define context.

Traditional software, non-ML, uses explicit index.

Machine Learning, Short for ML, uses implicit index.

Explicit index, uses static user-entered information,

To predict "1234" is a phone number as useful information.

Implicit index, uses dynamic machine-entered information,

to predict "1234" is a phone number as a useful information.

Both non-ML and ML software, encode and decode,

Meaningless data into meaningful information.

Implicit index in ML software, is quicker captured,

To explicit index in non-ML software capture.

But both has their own challenges.

ML software relies heavily on large data sets,

Non-ML software can consist of small data sets,

Wrong accuracy can happen in both cases if the data,

Transmitted is wrong for the wrong context.

In the digital realm where code and software intertwine,

Both non-ML and ML software strive to define,

Meaningless data into insights that shine,

The dance of encode and decode of data, in silicon shrine.

ML software, with its implicit index so keen,

Captures patterns quicker, in a computational dream.

Non-ML, with explicit index, does its part,

Though in smaller datasets, it finds its heart.

Yet, challenges lurk in both software path, so clear,

ML thirsts for vast data sets, a constant need to adhere.

Non-ML, though small in data sets, can still miss the mark,

If wrong context or data, into the digital system, does embark.

Accuracy, the goal, can be wrongly sung,

If the data fed, from the wrong context, has sprung.

In this digital quest for meaningful light,

Both kinds of software must handle data right.

Poem 4: Data mining

Data mining, digs deep,

Software tools, the ground they sweep.

Results like figs, ripe and sweet,

Knowledge harvested, no defeat.

Farmer with dig hoe, in the field,

Soil mining, secrets revealed.

Sunny days, soil turns to stone,

Hard to till, alone.

Rain comes pouring, softens the ground,

Soil covers all, without a sound.

Farmer uncovers, seeds to plant,

Soil covers back, as it wants.

New data flows, like a stream,

Machine learning, a data mining dream.

Uncovering patterns, hidden and deep,

In the digital world, where we reap,

As much as the farmer uncovers the soil heap.

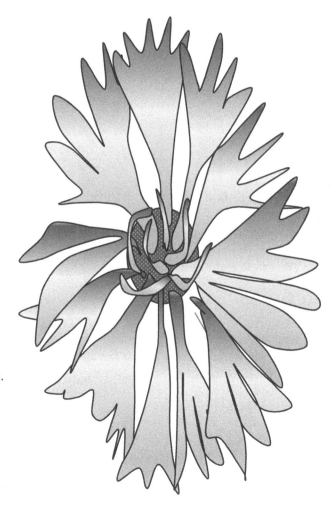

Poem 5: Data feeds

Datasets, a set of values,

quantitative or qualitative values.

1,2,3,4, as a large dataset,

More reliable onset,

Then 1,2 in a small dataset.

Having larger datasets,

avoid missing valuable asset,

an informational asset,

dispensable to a context.

Datasets increased,

Inhibit data feeds,

In Bulk or incrementally,

Existing data, layering

In multiple dimensions and directions,

With new data feeds addition

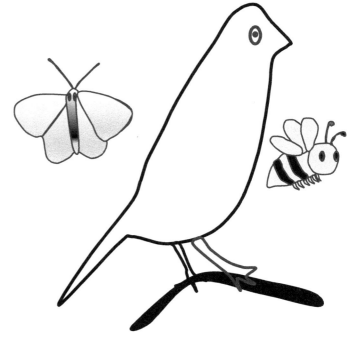

Hence, datasets when feeds,

Create a range of seeds,

As values to our deeds.

Poem 6: Mango & Machine Learning (ML)

The Mango tree mellow,

Acts as a vibrant tango.

Sometimes as a silent piano.

When it is windy, a tree tango,

Mangoes cascade down in the flow.

When it is sunny, a tree piano,

Mangoes defy time, ripening slow,

From green whispers to a yellowish glow.

Machine Learning, short for ML,

Similarly, acts as a vibrant tango,

Dancing through ML data with an insightful glow.

Sometimes as a silent piano,

It patiently learns, in a rhythmic echo,

Transforming raw knowledge into a powerful crescendo.

In the symphony of ML as a technology and nature,

Both perform their unique interlude,

One in the realm of the earthly crude,

The other in the digital universe's mood.

Together, they remind us of the intricate chance,

Between the natural world and human dance.

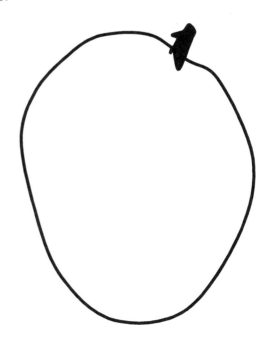

13

Poem 7: Apples & Machine Learning (ML)

Apples, in different colors,

Green, Red, often eye-catching pollars

White and Orange, often back to our collars,

The color varieties eye-daze us,

Little is known on these varieties' cases,

as a customer, visiting a fruit market place,

not self-questioning, but exploring its space,

another item to be chased and purchased,

fully occupied our mind base,

Machine Learning, short for ML,

Act like the fruit market,

ML decision makers alike human hamlet

Choose a data model like a fruit basket.

Data chosen, alike to apples chosen.

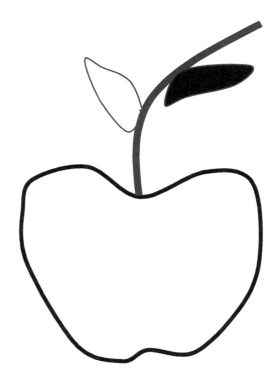

Apples differentiated by color characteristics,

Data, no colour characteristics.

Data, has situational linguistics,

With information in a style of artistic.

The varieties of these ML data,

different informational sources areas,

like apple trees triennial,

with grafted tree branch carriers.

A tree Grafting process,

a biological process,

produce, not less,

for sure, non-colourless apples.

Juicy, easily digest,

Farmer, grafting the scion,

From a branch, cut with precision,

Graft it to the rootstock,

Of a new tree, a fresh addition.

Scion, rootstock, buds, fusion,

Leads to apple colors, a diversion.

ML model, like the farmer,

Grafts, information as the scion,

From a different source, cut with precision

Graft it to the existing model progression,

As a fresh addition.

ML model, use fusion

to gather data in progression

Like the grafted tree passion,

To farm ML data, like apples

But Ml model, as outcome

To this fusion, outputs not some,

But one meaningful output,

For the Ml model sprouts,

Unlike the farmer, as outcome

To this fusion, outputs some

Beautiful apples

For the fruit market and customer

Poem 8: Oranges & Machine Learning (ML)

Florida in the United States trusties,

the Mediterranean countries,

Brazil, and parts of Asia mistiest,

All commonly, are hot regional sunnies.

These regions, best for some orange types,

Navel, Valencia oranges, keen to ripe.

In these regions, the citrus vitamin C thrives,

With ample sun and warm, moist lives.

The Navel, with its easy peel,

Its lack of seeds, a delight feel.

Valencia, its juice so sweet,

A late season treat, a citrus feat,

Memorable, not to quit.

These oranges, in their natural habitat,

Grow best in immense sunny areas.

Upon, unexpected cold, like in south Korea

The oranges, Navel, Valencia,

spoiled and turned into a yellowish feta,

Hard and cold, feta,

With a look of a thin tortilla.

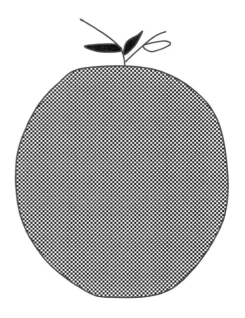

A slight change in temperature,

disastrous for the orange texture.

Great care required, as gesture

Windbreaks, smudge pots, awake solutions,

Row Covers, overhead sprinkles, inclusion,

Reduce the risk of oranges destruction,

When hot temperature, attrition.

In Machine Learning, short for ML,

The cold temperature attrition,

an ML outlier to the hot temperature seclusion.

Temperature outliers, identified by ML software,

Assist and speed farmers' solutions' care

Windbreaks, smudge pots, not spare

Row Covers, overhead sprinkles, there.

Poem 9: Grapes & Machine Learning (ML)

black, dark blue, yellow, green,

orange, pink, crimson colour beams

What are these?

The grapes variety gleams

But difficult to streamline,

When mixed, unordered and undivided.

Fortunately, wine production,

Either mixed or unmixed grapes, fusion,

Result into tasty composition.

In Machine Learning, short for ML,

Data are mixed, alike mixed grapes.

Stage 1, ML data collected,

Grapes harvested,

Carefully selected,

For data & grapes quality shed.

Stage 2, ML data cleaning,

Grape destemming and crushing,

Involves unwanted parts removing,

handling data values or grapes, missing.

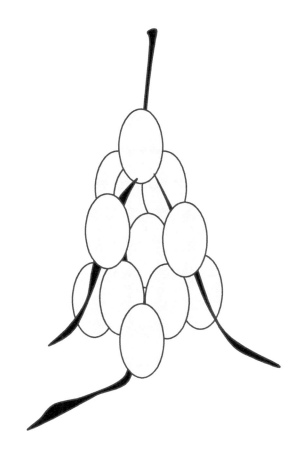

Stage 3, ML feature engineering,

Grape pressing.

Grape juice extracting,

Juice extracted affect wine aroma and flavour,

ML extract features from domain knowledge endeavour,

Yet, with the wrong ML extraction, predictions turn sour,

Mirroring wine poorly made, leaving a bitter dower.

Stage 4, ML data preprocessing,

Grape fermentation engineering,

Magical processes used for wine manufacturing,

Grape juice's sugars into alcohol non-drinking format,

Through yeast mixing.

ML pre-processed data, in a non-user format,

Alike the undrinking format of alcohol.

ML magical processes capped

From encoding categorical data to scaling,

and data normalization to produce this non-user format.

Stage 5, ML model training,

Over time, the process of Wine aging,

In stainless steel tanks or bottles, lingering.

Aroma and flavours, as time fingers.

ML let its training model perdure,

To grasp the data essence, its aroma and lure.

Recognition of data patterns, features it discerns,

Unveiling the trained model secrets, like the wine alcohol secrets turn.

Stage 6, ML evaluation, the process

of Wine quality control distribution,

Unforeseen ML data, test caption,

Unforeseen bad wines, test conformation.

Stage 7, ML model deployment,

Wine bottling enjoyment,

Include ready-to-sell wine agreement,

As much as ML model is ready-to-predict clement,

With purpose, a wine customer and a ML user, enjoyment

Stage 8, ML monitoring and updating,

A process mirroring the art of wine cellaring.

As wines evolve within the bottle,

So too does ML data require conditions to follow.

Just as wines need specific storage conditions to age with grace,

ML data can become outdated, requiring a new place.

Updates and monitoring ensure the model's relevance,

Much like the careful tending of a wine cellar's essence

Wine and machine learning (ML) share similarities,

For ML utilizes data as wine does grapes.

Both require careful selection and processing,

To yield results that are precise and crisp.

As wine is crafted from the essence of the vine,

ML models are built from data, piece by piece, fine.

Both are products of time, care, and expertise,

Creating experiences that delight and appease.

Poem 10: Pears & Machine Learning (ML)

Rosaceae, distinct family structure,

With flowers of five petals & sepals' sculpture,

The petals & sepals become part of the flower picture.

Rosaceae, include variety of fruits,

Apples from genetic genus Mulus,

Pears, from genetic genus Pyrus,

Cherries from genetic genus prenus.

Asteraceae, has no petal & sepal,

Are tiny flowers, the florets ornamental,

Lectuce, part of the family hierarchical,

Petals and sepals exist in monumental.

From genetic lactuca genus disposal,

Which produce lectuce as food special.

Lamiaceae has petals & sepals,

Genus, Genera in plural,

Produce aromatic leaves and flowers

Mints, rosemary, basil & lavenders,

To bestow for a nice dish to conquer.

For plants to grow,

Bear fruit at slow,

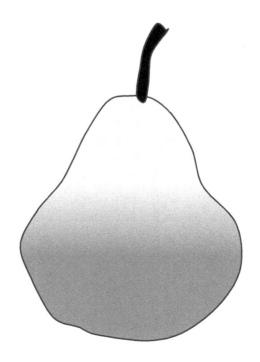

Water them to the toe.

In deep learning, a concept

In machine learning (ML), project,

Input, hidden and output layer.

In our plant examples, water are inputs

Output are the fruit or leaves,

Fruits as apple, pear

Leaves as mint, lavender

The hidden layer is mysterious fur.

In the neural network's depth, a mystery does unfold,

A hidden layer, where secrets manifold are told.

It consists of one or many input layers,

A realm of multi-perceptron, where true power layers.

The family structure, a 1st hidden input layer,

The Rosaceae family, inherits an ancestor so rare,

An ancestor with genetic divergence, a tale to share,

A 2nd hidden layer, where branches start to appear.

Genera Malus, for apples, in this layer does bloom,

Genera Pyrus, for pears, in the same genetic room.

Genera classification, a 3rd hidden layer, so astute,

Can be understood through morphological, genetic, and molecular loot.

Such hidden layers, create a multi-perceptron array,

In Machine Learning, a path to trace and convey.

To retrieve backward from the apple fruit, so sweet and round,

Its genetic composition, in these layers, we can find unbound.

Through the neural network's eye, we can see the past,

Unraveling the story of how species were cast.

In the depth of data, the truth we seek to find,

In the hidden layers, where ancestral links bind.

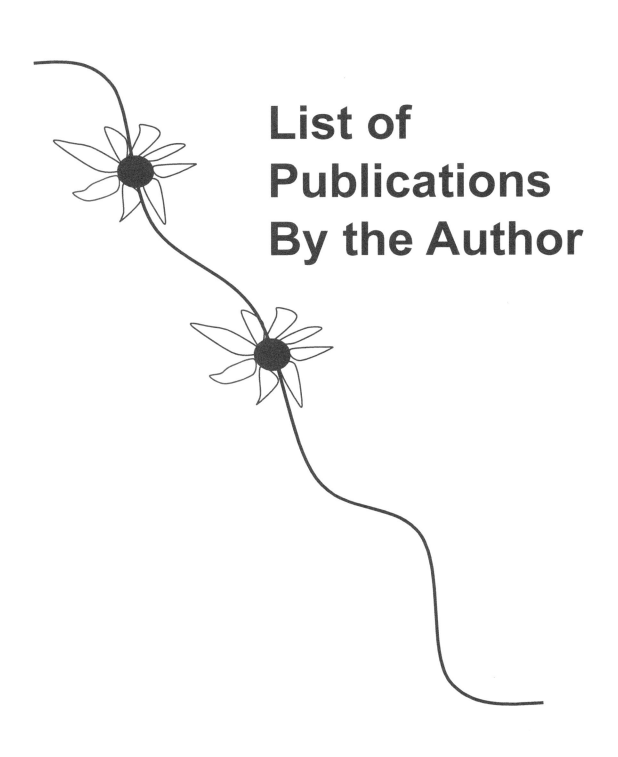

List of
Publications
By the Author

List of Journal/Conference Publications

Table 1 List of Academic publications by Yeeshtdevisingh Hosanee

	Book Title	Pub. Date	Age
1.	An enhanced software tool to aid novices in learning Object Oriented Programming (OOP)	2015	20+
2.	The need to teach object-oriented programming in undergraduate courses	2015	20+
3.	Using different assessment screens to evaluate students' Object-Oriented Programming (OOP) skills	2015	20+
4.	Is prior knowledge necessary for undergraduate computing courses? A study of courses offered by Mauritian universities	2015	20+
5.	The implementation of a 2 user proficiency level novice OOP software tool", published in Emergitech2016 conference (Mauritius) – published on	2016	20+
6.	Teaching English Literacy to Standard One Students: Requirements Determination for Remediation Through ICT, published in Emergitech2016 conference (Mauritius)	2016	20+
7.	The analysis and the need of ubiquitous learning to engage children in coding- published in 28-30 Nov 2018 conference	2018	20+
8.	Teaching an IT industry programming language to children of 10 years old-MRIC post-graduate conference 2020	2020	20+
9.	The Tabular API Testing Framework: used with JMeter and Microsoft Excel VBA	2021	20+

List of Book Publications

Table 2 List of book publications by Yeeshtdevisingh Hosanee

	Book Title	Pub. Date	Age	ISBN
1.	PYTHON IN ONE WEEK	2010	20+	Local book in Mauritius (co-author)
2.	APRAN PROGRAMMING DANS PYTHON (learn programming in Python, English version)	20/11/2021	10+	9789994908653
3.	Learn Python Programming	1/6/2022	10+	9789392274787
4.	Learn Java Programming	1/6/2022	10+	9789392274770
5.	Machine Learning: The 10 Classifiers In Python	17/8/2023	10+	9789392274893
6.	Artificial Intelligence: The 10 Examples In Python	17/8/2023	10+	9789392274558
7.	Artificial Intelligence - The Python Chatbot in Australia	18/3/2024	10+	9781923020566
8.	Diwali Celebration in Python	26/10/2024	8+	9789363555174
9.	Diwali Celebration in Python (French)	2/10/2024	8+	9789363553040
10.	Mother AI For This Christmas	11/11/ 2024	3+	9798346198673
11.	La mère ia pour ce noël : Les PREMIÈRS CONTES DE NOËL pour les enfants de 3+ ans À L'ÈRE DE L'INTELLIGENCE ARTIFICIELLE (AI)	2/11/ 2024	3+	9782322478620
12.	The Yeehos Tech-Poetry: My computer mimics My Badminton Players & Gardeners	12/11/ 2024	10+	9782322558339
13.	La fête des lumières en java (diwali): Les contes de Codage avec Crayon et du Papier pour les Enfants de 10+ Ans	2/11/2024	10+	9782322478859

www.ingramcontent.com/pod-product-compliance
Lightning Source LLC
LaVergne TN
LVHW082347060326
832902LV00016B/2704